1.

LOSING WEIGHT IS SIMPLE

Caloric Restriction Extends Lifespan

Losing Weight Made Simple

Lose Weight And Belly fat

Eat Less Live Long and Young

Increased Testosterone Levels

Intermittent Fasting recent Health Trend

Increased Human Growth Hormone, HGH

Dr. Arta Tran Dash, M.Sc., M. S., Ph. D.

Retired Professor

INTRODUCTION

Losing Weight is Simple

First thing you should do is to make a list what you usually eat. If the list contains any of the following foods, you must gradually stop eating them, if you can't stop eating them right away. Eat natural healthy foods. Below is the list of foods that I want you must avoid;

Grains, bread, cereal, wheat products, pasta, pizza, bagels, processed foods, processed meats, packaged foods, fast foods and fried foods, soda pops, energy drinks, juices (especially orange drink) and juice cocktail. I hope you got the message. If you stop taking these, you will see the changes within a week

your body did **not** evolve to consume starchy, high carbohydrate sugars from bread, pasta, cereal and other grains, soda pops, juice cocktails, energy drinks, etc . Ever since we were told to eat low fat, these foods have been the bulk of our diet

AS a result, there has been a modern epidemic of obesity and diabetes. At the same time, we face skyrocketing rates of dementia and Alzheimer's

Research shows a strong link between blood sugar disorders and every stage of dementia, starting from memory loss to mild cognitive impairment to Alzheimer's.

It is clear from above that diabetes is considered major risk for Alzheimer's. That's why Alzheimer's has been called **"Type 3 diabetes."**

Low Fat Craze: Forty years ago or so the low fat craze started which created health havoc, including obesity, diabetes, Alz's. This low fat craze gave rise to various unhealthy foods. Many companies new or old started producing artificial products----low fat this and low fat that, skim this and skim that, artificial egg products and artificial crab neat, diet this and diet that. These are all chemically laden foods, not natural; and seriously can cause harm to your health. Always eat natural foods.

Health Benefits Of Caloric Restriction

Ever since it was discovered that longevity gene Sirtuin switch was turned off at mother's womb, the researchers worked tirelessly to find ways to activate the longevity genes Sirtuins. Besides natural supplements, the simple process like caloric restriction (eating less or starving or fasting) activates the longevity genes Sirtuins. We will discuss these topics below in details.

A few things are necessary to mention first before we delve into the real issues.

- a drop in calorie extends your lifespan by 30 seconds

- One Soda pop lessens your lifespan by 4.6 years
- Recent study shows that Alzheimer disease is Type 3 diabetes
  This mean you need calorie restriction, especially coming from carbs
- Caloric restriction how important for health

Caloric restriction has numerous health benefits. As you have seen from above, it extends lifespan; because it activates the longevity genes Sirtuins. Would you believe, starvation or fasting activates longevity genes sirtuins. It also activates intelligent gene BDNF which makes you smart and mentally alert. It increases production of **Human Growth Hormone** (HGH), helps you lose belly fat and lose weight. See later for details.

Healh Benefits of Eating Less:

Eating less not only activates the longevity gene **Sirtuin 1** (SIRT 1), and other SIRTs, but also many other health benefits. Live long and feel smart, Improved mood, sleep, sex drive, and blood sugar levels, feel alert and energetic, lose weight and belly fat, look and feel young, keep you slim and handsome, feel good about yourself, become smarter, and reduced cholesterol level and high blood pressure, improved heart and brain health, disease free. Cutting back on food repairs all your organs in the body. You save money, and extend your lifespan

The single most important health improving, life changing thing you can do to transform your diet to eat more vegetables. Numerous studies have shown that those who eat all or mostly vegetables have better quality of life. A growing body of scientific evidences suggests that the regular consumption of diet rich in vegetables and fruits reduce the risk of chronic diseases, increase lifespan and quality of life

What Is Intermittent Fasting?

As you have noted fasting has numerous health benefits. Many religions, such as Hinduism, Buddhism, and Christianity practice religious fasting. If you have been eating for 49 or 60 or 70 years, all your organs are working relentlessly for digestion and absorption of foods, and transport the nutrients to different parts of the body. They never had any rest. Now fasting occasionally once or twice a week for 24 hours will give these organs time to repair and rejuvenate them. Sometimes, it is not plausible to do 24 hours fasting. However, there is a very popular and healthy method known as intermittent fasting. Popular method is 16/8.

Very simply 16/8 method mean 16 hours fast with 8 hour window. That is don't eat anything after dinner until lunch. a 16–hour fast followed by an 8–hour eating period.

Caution:

Intermittent fasting is certainly not for everyone.

If you are underweight, or have a history of eating disorders, then you should not do intermittent fasting without consulting with a healthcare professional first.

In these cases, it can be very harmful.

For women, it is not advisable to do intermittent fasting. It is not beneficial for women. Moreover, women who are trying to be pregnant or pregnant or nursing should not do intermittent fasting.

LOKA SAMASTA SUKHINO BHABANTU

(Let Each And Every Person In The Universe Be Hale and Hearty)

VEDAS

DEDICATION

This book is dedicated to the memory of my father (Linga Raj Dash) and my Mother (Mukta Debi) whose unconditional love nurtured my life through and through. It is also dedicated to all those who read it, use it, and benefit from it.

DISCLAIMER

This book is not intended to diagnose, treat or replace the service of a doctor. If you have any health conditions or are under a doctor's care, you must consult your physician or a healthcare

professional before you apply any of the recommendations set forth in the pages of this book.

All information available in this book is for educational purposes only, and none of the stated products have been FDA approved. Any application of the recommendations mentioned in this book is at the readers' discretion and sole risk.

The publication is offered "as is" without warranty of any kind either expressed or implied, including but not limited to, the implied warranties of merchantability, suitability for a particular purpose or non-infringement. Descriptions of or reference to products or publications does not imply endorsement of that product or publication.

Here is how you can use the information in this book to improve your health and wellness. Being Empowered with these powerful armies of information, and the knowledge gathered from it, you would be able to discuss your health problems with a healthcare professional and design a regimen that is conducive to your health and well being, instead of just being drugged to death and suffer from lethal side effects of these drugs, causing serious debilitating, chronic diseases, even death.

If you find your physician is unwilling to discuss the issue, find another physician or a healthcare professional who is more sensitive to your wish and willing to take the time to listen to you for your well being. You need to know all your options before embarking on a particular regimen or a procedure.

TABLE OF CONTENTS

Blood sugar levels

Lose weight and belly fat

Look and feel young

Improved heart and brain health

Repairs all your organs

Nutritional Ketosis

Carbohydrates

Intermittent fasting

CHAPTER THREE

Carbohydrates are two types; **complex carbohydrates** and **simple carbohydrates**

Complex carbohydrates

Simple carbohydrates

Barley and oatmeal

Black beans

Processed foods

Soda pops

Fiber

Antioxidant compounds

Anthocyanins

CHAPTER FOUR

Healthy fats are **Monounsaturated fats** and **Polyunsaturated fats**

Monounsaturated fats:

Avocado

Extra virgin olive oil

Extra virgin coconut oil

Nuts: almonds, peanuts, hazelnuts, pecans, Brazil nuts, walnuts

Polyunsaturated fats:

Sunflower seeds, sesame seeds, and their oils but don't cook with it,

Don't take canola oil

Walnut, sunflower

Salmon, tuna, mackerel, trout, herring, sardines

Omega -3

Saturated fats

Meats, poultry, ghee

Diabetes

Trans Fats

LDL cholesterol

HDL cholesterol

Hydrogenated vegetable oils

Fried foods

Margarine

Processed and package foods

CHAPTER FIVE

PROTEIN

Red meat, poultry, seafood, beans, lentils

Ounce, grams

Lose weight

Fruits and vegetables

Fed sate

Fasted state

Gynostemma

CHAPTER EIGHT

Intermittent Fasting May Cure Diabetes

Diabetes

Metformin

Risk of cancer

Slow aging process

Feast and famine

Pancreas cells

Beta cells

Type 1 and Type 2 diabetes

16/8 method

INTRODUCTION

Losing Weight is Simple

First thing you should do is to make a list what you usually eat. If the list contains any of the following foods, you must gradually stop eating them, if you can't stop eating them right away. Eat natural healthy foods. Below is the list of foods that I want you must avoid;

Grains, bread, cereal, wheat products, pasta, pizza, bagels, processed foods, processed meats, packaged foods, fast foods and fried foods, soda pops, energy drinks, juices (especially orange drink) and juice cocktail. I hope you got the message. If you stop taking these, you will see the changes within a week

your body did ***not*** evolve to consume starchy, high carbohydrate sugars from bread, pasta, cereal and other grains, soda pops, juice cocktails, energy drinks, etc . Ever since we were told to eat low fat, these foods have been the bulk of our diet

AS a result, there has been a modern epidemic of obesity and diabetes. At the same time, we face skyrocketing rates of dementia and Alzheimer's

Research shows a strong link between blood sugar disorders and every stage of dementia, starting from memory loss to mild cognitive impairment to Alzheimer's.

It is clear from above that diabetes is considered major risk for Alzheimer's. That's why Alzheimer's has been called **"Type 3 diabetes."**

Low Fat Craze: Forty years ago or so the low fat craze started which created health havoc, including obesity. This low fat craze gave rise to various unhealthy foods. Many companies new or old started producing artificial products----low fat this and low fat that, skim this and skim that, artificial egg products and artificial crab neat, diet this and diet that. These are all chemically laden foods, not natura; and seriously cause harm to your health. Always eat natural foods, and consider natural to your ailments if any..

CHAPTER ONE

Health Benefits Of Caloric Restriction

Ever since it was discovered that longevity gene Sirtuin switch was turned off at mother's womb, the researchers worked tirelessly to find ways to activate the longevity genes Sirtuins. Besides natural supplements, the simple process like caloric restriction (eating less or starving or fasting) activates the longevity genes Sirtuins. We will discuss these topics below in details.

A few things are necessary to mention first before we delve into the real issues.

- a drop in calorie extends your lifespan by 30 seconds
- One Soda pop lessens your lifespan by 4.6 years
- Recent study shows that Alzheimer disease is Type 3 diabetes
  This mean you need calorie restriction, especially coming from carbs
- Caloric restriction how important for health

Caloric restriction has numerous health benefits. As you have seen from above, it extends lifespan; because it activates the longevity genes Sirtuins. Would you believe, starvation or fasting activates longevity genes sirtuins. It also activates intelligent gene BDNF which makes you smart and mentally alert. It increases production of **Human Growth Hormone** (HGH), helps you lose belly fat and lose weight. See later for details.

CHAPTER TWO

How Does One Achieve Caloric Restriction?

There are three different methods that will help you consume fewer calories, for instance eating less, starving or fasting, as mentioned above.

Eating Less has many health benefits. Consume more fats and moderate amounts of proteins (excess protein will trigger cancer cells), less carbs (carb:fat:protein = 40%:35%:25%, make sure you get these carbs more from vegetables and moderately from fruits).

Health Benefits of Eating Less:

Eating less not only activates the longevity gene **Sirtuin 1** (SIRT 1), and other SIRTs, but also many other health benefits. Live long and feel smart, Improved mood, sleep, sex drive, and blood sugar levels, feel alert and energetic, lose weight and belly fat, look and feel young, keep you slim and handsome, feel good about yourself, become smarter, and reduced cholesterol level and high blood pressure, improved heart and brain health, disease free. Cutting back on food repairs all your organs in the body. You save money, and extend your lifespan

- Slower rate cell divisions
- The rate of glycation drops
- Reduced free radical activity
- Reduced inflammation

The single most important health improving, life changing thing you can do to transform your diet to eat more vegetables. Numerous studies have shown that those who eat all or mostly vegetables have better quality of life. A growing body of scientific evidences suggests that the regular consumption of diet rich in vegetables and fruits reduce the risk of chronic diseases, increase lifespan and quality of life.

Nutritional Ketosis: when you eat healthy high good fats (60 to 70 %), low carbs (10 to 5 %, from vegetables) and low to-moderate protein (30 to 25 %) diet your body enters into a state where body burns fats from your body as its primary fuel rather than glucose (sugar). Nutritionists call this state as **Nutritional Ketosis.** A growing body of scientific evidence suggests nutritional ketosis is the answer to a long list of health problems, including **obesity.** With low carb, high fat,- moderate amount of protein the insulin (fat storing hormone) is low leading to weight loss.

You may be careful to avoid all the sources of carbohydrates (sugar, sweets, bread, pasta, rice, potatoes, juices, juice cocktails, energy drinks, soda pops, you got the point), but if you are eating a large amount of meat, eggs, and the like, the excess protein will convert into glucose in the body. The large amount of protein can increase your insulin level somewhat leading to weight gain. This compromises the healthful effects of ketosis.

Numerous research studies indicates that nutritional ketosis has many applications, relating to heart health, seizure, diabetes, neurological disorders like Alzheimer's, Parkinson's, and cancer is another area, it is showing some promise. High fat diet helps starve cancer cells. Without glucose cancer cells will starve to death.

Intermittent Fasting (IF): It is not always plausible to starve or fast. But there are certain types of fasting one can do that will bring numerous health benefits. A popular one is called **intermittent fasting**. The combination of eating less and intermittent fasting, together gives rise to numerous health benefits, including weight loss and loss of belly fat. Before we discuss intermittent fasting, you need to know about carbohydrates, fats, and proteins.

CHAPTER THREE

Carbohydrates are two types; **complex carbohydrates** and **simple carbohydrates.**

What are Carbohydrates (Carbs)?

Most of us equate carbs with bread, rice, wheat, pasta baggies, cakes, and muffins, but you can find them in almost everything, vegetables, fruits, dairy prods, ucts, grains (wheat, rice, quinoa, Kamet, Barley). Sugar and Sugary products, and sweets, acorn squash, dairy products, they are all considered carbohydrates. We get calories from carbs, fats and proteins.

Complex carbs consist of whole grains, starchy vegetables, oatmeal, brown rice, Quinoas, oatmeal, barley, Kamut, legumes (peas, beans, green peas, and lentils), nuts and seeds. These are some of the examples of complex carbohydrates. Kamut contains 20 % magnesium. All the nuts and seeds contain magnesium.

Barley: is good for health. Reduce cholesterol, decreased blood sugar and increased satiety. Tons of health benefits like decreased inflammation, stabilized blood sugar, help regulate bowel movement.

Oatmeal: helps to lose weight, stabilizes blood sugar levels, boosts energy and heart health, lowers high blood pressure and cholesterol, lowers risk of colon cancer, and many more.

Black Beans : all beans are good for heart, but none can boost your brain power like black beans, because they contain anthocyanins, and antioxidant compounds that have been shown to improve brain function

Simple Carbs: fruits, vegetables, low fat diary, less nutritionally dense are sugar, sugary products, refined grains like white bread, white rice, processed foods and snacks, crackers, sweets, and cakes, soda pops, and juices. 1 slice of bread contains 30 grams of carbs and at least 3 grams of fiber

CHAPTER FOUR

HEALTHY FATS

Healthy fats are **monounsaturated fats** and **polyunsaturated fats**

Monounsaturated Fats: avocado (Buying Tip: buy organic unripe avocado and place them in a brown paper bag until the flesh appears a bit soft , then place them in fridge or eat one of them put rest in fridge,) olive oil (buying tip: there a lot of olive oils are adulterated with vegetable oils. Buy extra virgin olive oil EVOO.

If you are buying France olive oil look for AOC logo, from Italy DOP logo, from Spain DO logo, For California olive oil look for logo "COOC." Extra virgin coconut oil is extremely healthy for health. Take at least a little over two tablespoon extra virgin coconut oil every day. Take also MCT oil. You will also get monounsaturated fats from the following.

Nuts: Almonds, peanuts, Macadamia nuts, Hazelnuts, pecans, not cashew,

Polyunsaturated Fats

You can get it from consuming Safflower, Sesame, and Sunflower seeds and their oils. You can't use these oils for cooking. They get oxidized in high heat and become harmful to health. Oils such as corn oil, canola oil are not good for health. The following foods will also replenish you with polyunsaturated fats.

Walnuts, Sunflower, Sesame, pumpkin seeds, Tofu, soy milk (my advice would be not to take any soya products for two reasons, they have some serious side effects and they are also 99 % GMO.)

Fat fish, such as salmon, tuna, mackerel, trout, herring, sardines.

Do not take fish which are firm raised. Look for lable wild not farm raised

Edamame is both poly and mono unsaturated.

Take Full fat yogurt and full fat milk, if you intend to take them. Do not take skim milk or low fat yogurt, low fat dairy products, since all the essentials of milk has been taken out, what's left are additives, chemicals, sugar, and so on. It is not very healthy. This will make you obese and cause chronic diseases.

Omega-3 (krill oil or fish oil) fatty acids and omega-6 (vegetable oils) fatty acids.

This low taf and skim business have been causing serious health problems. It is a big business now, producing many unhealthy products for market. This has made people obese and has caused cardiovascular diseases

Saturated Fat:

This type fats come from animal sources of foods like meat, poultry, and full fat dairy products, ghee. It raises cholesterol levels LDL, bad cholesterol), also increase the risk of diabetes. Excessive intake of these foods may trigger cancer cells.

Trans Fat: Trans fats raise the LDL (bad) cholesterol levels and lowers the HDL (good) cholesterol levels. Variety of food products made using hydrogenated vegetable oils contain trans fats. For instance, baked goods (cakes, cookies, and crackers), potato, corn, tortilla chips, fried foods, creamer and margarine, processed and packaged foods. These foods are extremely harmful to health.

HEALTH BENEFITS OF COCONUT OIL

For years, coconut fat was demonized as the enemy of heart health — until multiple studies revealed that it's chock full of antioxidants and vitamin E. It also contains a unique kind of fat called medium-chain triglycerides, or MCTs — and these are extremely good for your heart.

You may also know that coconuts can:

- Help prevent obesity by speeding up your metabolism;
- It can reverse or cure Alz's disease. See below
- Help reduce high cholesterol and increase HDL (good) cholesterol levels
- Prevents heart disease and high blood pressure
- Improve brain function and memory
- Provide a quick energy boost;

- Reduce sugar cravings;
- Help prevent diabetes by improving insulin efficiency;
- Promote healthy thyroid function;
- Cures urinary track infection, kidney infection, and protects the liver
- Improve symptoms and inflammatory conditions associated with digestive and bowel disorders;
- Support your immune system;
- Improve antibacterial, anti-fungal, and anti-viral
- Increase energy and insurance
- Improve digestion, reduce stomach ulcers, and ulcerative colitis
- Cancer prevention and treatment
- Reduce inflammation and arthritis
- Reduce symptoms of gallbladder disease and pancreatitis
- Help prevent type II diabetes
- Prevent osteoporosis
- Break up blood clots;
- Moisturizes and protects skin;
- Repairs dry damaged hair.

Coconuts are also hypoallergenic, and they contain antibacterial, antiviral and anti-parasitic healing properties.

Coconut oil contains medium-chain fatty acids that help improve thyroid functioning. It will also stimulate metabolism and boost energy. Plus, it will help raise the **basal body temperature** which is important for those dealing with low thyroid function.

A medical doctor cure her **husband's Alzheimer** disease by giving him a little over two and half tablespoons of coconut oil every morning http://healthiertalk.com/coconut-oil-as-an-alzheimers-treatment?utm_source=HealthierTalk&utm_medium=subemail&utm_campaign=Alzheimers_15.06.19

*But now researchers have discovered what traditional cultures have known for centuries: Coconut is a powerful anti-fungal treatment — especially against common yeast infections, like **Candida albicans**.*

Recommendation: add a few tablespoons of this oil to your existing diet to naturally manage any yeast infections. Look for virgin, unrefined coconut oil in your health food store. I recommend adding two to three tablespoons of coconut oil to your daily diet. You may use it in soup or curry, salads, etc.

For most recipes, you can simply add an equal amount of coconut oil in place of butter, margarine or shortening.

- Use coconut oil instead of butter in your cookies and cakes. Not only will you get the delicious flavor, but most of the fat you'll be eating will get burned off right away.
- Use it in place of oil when you sauté. Coconut oil has a high smoke point so it won't degrade at high temperatures. Other oils (even olive oil0 have low smoke point get oxidized at high temperature causing chronic diseases.
- Scoop a serving of coconut oil into a smoothie or bake it into snack bars for a healthy, delicious dose on the road.

CHAPTER FIVE

Protein

Proteins are found in meat, fish, poultry, eggs, legume, nuts and seeds.. Below you will get a general idea of protein content in various foods. Dr. Mercola.

-   Red meat, poultry and seafood, contain average 6 to 9 grams of protein per ounce. An ideal amount per serving of meat or seafood would be 3 to 5 ounce (not 9 or 12 ounce of steak) which will provide 18 to 27 grams of protein.

-   Seeds and nuts contain an average of 4 to 8 grams of proteins per quarter cup;
    Cooked grains contain 5 t0 7 grams of protein per cup

-   One egg contains 6 to 8 grams of protein,

-   Cooked beans on average contains 7 to 8 grams per a half cup

-   Most vegetables contain 1 to 2 grams of proteins per ounce

    .   Unit: 1 ounce = 28.35.. Grams

    .   1 gram of fat contains 9 calories

    .   Carbohydrate and protein each contains 4 calories per gram

    .   As you see calories come from carbs, fats, and proteins. If you eat more calories than   body needs, you will Gain weight. On the other hand, if you eat fewer calories than   required, you will lose weight.

If you intend to lose weight 1 lb per week, you should restrict your calorie consumption to 1600 --1800 per day; and with the proportion of carbs (technically carbs are not essential to your diet, since body can get fuel from fat and protein), fat, as follows: .

Get All The Carbs From Vegetables and Fruits Rather Than Grains and Beans.

If you want to lose more than 1 lb a week, then restrict your calorie consumption to somewhere in between1600 to 1800 calorie per day.

Fed State when body is digesting and absorbing foods It takes three to five hours. During this period it is very hard for body to burn fat, because insulin your insulin levels are high. After four or five hours, the body goes to

fasted state. It is much easier for body to burn fat in fasted state because your insulin level is low. In fasted state your body burns just body fat as primary fuel, thereby it helps lose weight. Thus, fasting puts the body in fat burning state that you rarely make it to during your normal eating cycle.

CHAPTER SIX

What Is Internet Fasting?

As you have noted fasting has numerous health benefits. Many religions, such as Hinduism, Buddhism, and Christianity practice religious fasting. If you have been eating for 49 or 60 or 70 years, all your organs are working relentlessly for digestion and absorption of foods, and transport the nutrients to different parts of the body. They never had any rest. Now fasting occasionally once or twice a week for 24 hours will give these organs time to repair and rejuvenate them. Sometimes, it is not plausible to do 24 hours fasting. However, there is a very popular and healthy method known as intermittent fasting.

Intermittent Fasting is currently is one of the world's most popular health and fitness trends. People are using it to lose weight and belly fat; improve their healthy life style and have longer life. Numerous studies reported that IF can have powerful impacts on your body and brain, and help you live longer; reduce risk of cancer.

Intermittent fasting involves 16 hours fasting or fasting for 24 hours twice a week. We all fast everyday while we sleep. For intermittent fasting just extend this fast a little longer. You can do this by skipping breakfast, eating first meal at noon and your last meal at 8 PM. This is popularly known as 16/8 method. This means you are restricting your eating to an 8 hour eating window. This is the most popular form of intermittent fasting known as 16/8 method, 8 hour window in eating.

Intermittent fasting is fairly easy to do, and it is easier than dieting. Many people have reported feeling better, having more energy, and mentally alert, even during fast. Food only takes 4 hours for digestion. After that the body is in fasted state. During that state body initiates important repair processes and changes the gene expressions. Health benefits of IF;

- lose weight and belly fat
- insulin levels drops and hence improved fat burning
- lower blood cholesterol levels
- lower blood insulin levels and blood sugar levels
- insulin levels drop dramatically, making the stored fat accessible for use as primary fuel for energy. This leads to weight loss
- Can Reduce Insulin Resistance, Lowering Your Risk of Type 2 Diabetes
- reversal of Type-2 diabetes
- improved heart and brain health
- prevention of Alzheimer disease (Type-3 diabetes)
- activates longevity gene SIRTs which leads to longer life
- Human Growth Hormone (HGH) skyrockets, increasing as much as 5-fold
- Increased energy
- Activates the intelligent gene BDNF (Brain Derived Neurotrophic Factor) that makes you smarter
- Improved mental clarity and concentration
- Reduction of inflammation
- Activation of cellular cleansing. In fasted state, you cells initiate processes where cells digest and remove old and dysfunctional proteins that buildup inside the cells
- Activates longevity genes SIRTs leading to long life
- Activates enzyme AMPK that has numerous health benefits including weight loss, flat belly, and fertility in both sexes. It is the potent fat burner. See details below.

CHAPTER SEVEN

ENZYME AMPK

Enzyme AMPK (Adenosine monophosphate-activated protein kinase) is in every cell in your body. AMPK serves as your cells master regulating switch, when activated or turned on that would burn fat and turn up your metabolism. It plays a vital role in determining your body fat composition. When you are young AMPK is more active, but as you age the cellular AMPK activation decreases leading to fat accumulation and decreased muscle mass.

Fortunately, certain dietary planning and food components greatly improve AMPK activity. As a result, these natural strategies hold great promise in the pursuit of near effortless weight loss.

- **Caloric restriction activates AMPK**
  fewer than 1200 caloric may help activate AMPK
- **Intermittent Fasting activates AMPK**
- **Overeating inhibits AMPK activity and**
- **AMPk is decreased in Overweight individuals**
- **High intensity exercise significantly increases AMPK activity**

BELLY FAT and AMPK:

Not all body fats are same. Certain types like **abdominal fat** pose the greatest danger to health. Abdominal fat not only unattractive, but also life threatening; and can speed up the aging process. Deep abdominal fat generates massive inflammatory chemicals that attack your body and produce more fat starting a vicious cycle that needs targeted intervention.

These inflammatory chemicals cause serious degenerative disorders that include dementia, diabetes, cardiovascular disease, reduced blood flow, high blood pressure, heart attacks, strokes, certain cancers, and potential bone and joint deterioration.

Scientists discovered that blood vessels of an individual with large abdominal fat deposits are deficient in **nitric oxide,** the signaling molecule that tells arteries to relax and dilate, and improving blood flow and blood pressure. During their investigation they discovered that **boosing AMPK** resulted in an unprecedented effects – **the reduction of abdominal fat.**

A process by which the cells "clean house or toxic cellular debris" is called **autophagy.** This is how cells remove damaged proteins, dysfunctional mitochondria, viruses, and other metabolic waste products. Research indicates that when **autophagy** diminished, the premature aging accelerates. Thus, it is imperative to restore healthy autophagy to slow and reverse biological aging.

Research also showed that by activating or boosting **AMPK** leads to following benefits:

- increased autophagy -- slow biological aging, and result in longer life
- activated AMPK signals cells to remove internal pollutants
- helping cells to remove debris via AMPK activation may result in reduced belly fat

- activation of AMPK leads to reduced inflammation and other damage it wreaks

Prescription drug metformin can boost AMPK activation, but it may have side effects. Here we will just mention two natural ingredients, **hesperidin** and **Gynostemma pentaphyllum** extract. Below you will find a whole list of ingredients that activate AMPK.

HESPERIDIN

Hesperidin is found primarily in citrus fruits and is classified as a "bioflavonoid." Hesperidin is known to have beneficial effects on blood vessels. It is touted as a natural remedy for a slew of health problems, including allergies, hemorrhoids, high blood pressure, hot flashes, hay fever, varicose veins, and premenstrual syndromes Neutralizes free radical reactive oxygen species, helps reduce the incidence of cancer in rats. It is anti-inflammatory. Hesperidin protects heart and brain. It controls blood sugar and may lower cholesterol. **It also helps fat loss**.

It has a number of side effects, including abdominal pain, diarrhea, and lowers blood pressure, not good for people who have low blood pressure, clinical research indicates that hesperidin may affect blood clotting and increase the risk of bleeding. People going for surgery should stop taking hesperidin two weeks before and two weeks after. If you have blood dis orders, you must consult with your doctor before taking hesperidin.

Gynostemma

Health Benefits

- Gynostema is considered herb of immortality in China.
- It is also considered poor man's ginseng. It contains 80 different saponins compared to 28 found in ginseng--- making it to be considered as steroid on ginseng
- **Heart Health:** according to the study by Vanderbilt University—gynostemma contains one of the saponins that facilitates the release of nitric oxide by the blood vessels. This in turn causes them to relax, leading to increased blood flow, thus lowering high blood pressure and decreasing the risk of athersclerosis.
- The study also found that this herb has blood thinning properties, reducing the aggregation of blood platelets and ameliorating the buildup of plaque.
- Energy: The Chinese have traditionally drunk tea made from jiaogulan to give them the energy that they need throughout a hard day of labor.
- In case your immune system is compromised, gynostemma can boost your immune system to fight against bacteria, viruses, parasites, and fungi sicknesses ranging from common colds, flu to cancer
- **WEIGHT LOSS:** One clinical study published in 2006 actually showed that it could help people with fatty liver disease and also help reduce their body mass index. (5) **(5)** http://www.ncbi.nlm.nih.gov/pubmed/16708768
- Anti-aging, anti- cancer potential, improves diabetes and blood sugar, good for the skin

Gynostemma side effects

JIAOGULAN (another name for gynostemma) Side Effects & Safety. Jiaogulan is POSSIBLY SAFE when taken by mouth short-term (up to **4 months**). In some people, it may cause side effects **like severe** nausea and increased bowel movements.

Precautions and Side Effects:

Gynostemma should not be taken with any medicine or herbs that affect blood clotting or immune system suppression.

Do not take when pregnant or nursing without first discussing with your doctor.

Do not this product when you are pregnant since it can always lead to possible birth defects once the baby is born.

Other possible side effects are:

- The "Auto-immune diseases" like multiple sclerosis (MS)
- lupus (systemic lupus erythematosus, SLE)
- rheumatoid arthritis (RA)

Gynostemma can aggravate and increase these symptoms of the autoimmune diseases. When you have an autoimmune condition you should not use the product since it comes with many other side effects like bleeding disorders from a slowed down blood clotting process. This may also make this bleeding disorder even worse if measures are not taken.

People undergoing for surgery should avoid gynostemma

Read Original Article: http://www.herbslist.net/gynostemma.html

Health Benefits Of AMPK Activation:

AMPK Helps with fertility in both sexes by increasing the production of sex hormones, it is the potent fat burner, holds near effortless fat loss, helps revitalize aging cells and promote new mitochondria (the power house of cells), promotes healthy aging and extends lifespan by 20 to 30 percent, inhibits multiple damaging factors associate with aging, activating AMPK may help multiple longevity pathways to promote healthy aging, decrease inflammation, improves diabetes, protects heart, prevents cancer, increases testosterone levels.

When AMPK is increased the body kicks into high gear and functions with youthful vitality

Following Natural Supplements That can Activate AMPK

Quercetin, berberine, gynostemma from jiaogulan, Trans-tiliroside from rose hips, curcumin, resveratrol, anthocyanins (blueberries, bilberries, grape seed extracts, pine bark extract [pycnogenol]), fish oil, panax ginseng, astralgus, mulberry leaf extract, Nootkatone, green coffee bean extract, DHA and EPA, extra virgin olive oil, extra virgin coconut oil, ACV, green tea (EGCG), Rooibus tea (do not use milk or sugar, just boiled water). Polyphenol (red grapes, blueberries, or berries in general), hot peppers, cayenne peppers, capsaicin, can activate AMPK or are fat burning foods.

The most promising AMPK activator is Jiaogulan (Gynostemma).

Health Benefits of Jiaogulan:

Lowers Homoglobin A1c
Lowers triglycerides
Improves insulin sensitivity
Reduces liver inflammation
Promotes weight loss
Neuroprotective effect
Activates AMPK

Jiaogulan can be drunk as a tea, as a liquid extract, or taken as a concentrated extract in capsules. The standard dose is 450 mg daily. It is non-toxic so can be used for several months without adverse effects.

NOTE: the effects of intermittent fasting are nullified if you binge on foods after fasting periods. You still have to keep portion low, that is, **EAT LESS. Get** Carbs from Vegetables and Fruits rather than grains, include healthy fats, that is, low carbs (from vegetable and fruits), low protein, and high in healthy fats.

CHAPTER EIGHT

Intermittent Fasting May Cure Diabetes

When you are diagnosed as having diabetes, your doctor will put you on a drug called metformin. This drug can cause serious side effects like dizziness, fatigue, cardiovascular reactions, flu like symptoms, , muscle pain, diarrhea and anemia.

As I mentioned above, intermittent fasting currently is one of the world's most popular health and fitness trends. People are using it to lose weight and belly fat. Studies show that it has powerful impact on your body and mind, and can help you live longer, make you smarter, reduce your risk of cancer.

As you have seen from above that IF triggers powerful health benefits and even slows down the aging process.

Recently, in an exciting research study, researchers from University of Southern California have found that **Intermittent Fasting** -- which mimics the ancient primal life style of "feast and famine" --- can turn around both type 1 and type 2 diabetes.

" Feast and Famine" means often your primal ancestors went for long periods of time with very little foods—at least until the next successful hunt. But these extended periods of hunger did not damage their bodies rather it regenerated them.

Now scientists have discovered that intermittent fasting also triggers the regeneration of key pancreas cells.

This is great news in the fight against diabetes.

You know, your pancreas produces hormone insulin that controls your blood sugar levels.

Previous groundbreaking research from USC showed that intermittent fasting makes stem cells to awaken from their normal dormant state and begin regenerating. And the latest study reveals that's exactly what happens in your pancreas.

USC researchers mimicking 'feast and famine" diet kick started a special type of cell in the pancreas called a ***beta cell.*** These are the cells that identify sugar in the blood and release insulin if it gets too high.

By regenerating pancreas beta cells, the researchers were able to restore mice from type 1 diabetes and late stage type 2 diabetes.

They also reactivated insulin production in human pancreatic cells from type 1 diabetes patients.

USC researchers used a modified version of the ancient feast and famine diet --- a low calorie, low protein, low carbohydrates, but high fat to regenerate the insulin producing pancreatic cells.

The human equivalent of this diet contains about 800 to 1,100 calories a day for five days with lots of nuts and soups. Then they allowed 25 days of normal eating---thus, overall it mimics ancient time of feast and famine.

There are various forms of fasting people practice. People fast two days at a time every month. Most popular method now a days is the 16/8 method discussed above. After your body gets used to 16/8 method, you can move up to 24 hours fasting or fast one days a week or two days at a time in a month. However, my advise— stick to 16/8 method, which is simpler.

USE FOODS TO GET FLAT BELLY

- **start the morning**
  with a cup of ginger tea that will stimulate your sluggish digestive system and increase your metabolic rate. Boil tbsp of grated ginger with a 1 ½ cup of water and your favorite tea bag (green tea or peppermint tea)

- **Eat a banana.**
  Bananas are packed with potassium that aids in flpuid balance to flatten belly bloat

- **Load on Cilantro** (coriander)
  Has a unique blend of oils (linalool and geranyl acetate) work to relax digestive muscles and alleviate an overactive gut. Study showed that patients with IBS relieve their symptoms supplementing with coriander

- **Dark chocolate:**
  Make sure dark chocolate contains at least cocoa content 70% or above. Beneficial microbes in our gut convert the dark chocolate into anti-inflammatory compounds which is beneficial to heart. When the

cocoa in dark chocolate reaches stomach's digestive juices and enzymes, the good microbes in the gut ferment it into anti-inflammatory compounds: you lose belly bloat.

- **Don't eat foods**

  that are greasy. Foods that are high in grease or are really fatty, like a McDonald's breakfast, can cause gastrointestinal upset. While some fats are good like coconut oil, olive oil, and omega-3 fatty acids good for health, nut fast foods contain unhealthy and harmful fats like saturated fats, trans fats that cause inflammatory response in the body, and chronic degenerative diseases.

- **Eat slowly so you don't gulf air:**

  eating too quickly or gulping food in a hurry causes you to swallow excess air, which can lead to uncomfortable gas and bloating. It is understandable that after a long day of work you are totally famished---it makes you to gulp food down. May be you should have a handful of nuts or seeds on your way home. Then after you settle down, sit down and have a leisurely supper.

- **Cut out diary see how you feel**

  Diary can be very cumbersome to belly, because as we get older our production of required digestive enzyme lactase declines. If you consume diary products pretty regularly, try cutting them out for a few days and see how your body reacts.

- **Take probiotic,**

  this will increase beneficial bacteria in the gut, needed for healthy gut. Gut is not healthy nothing will be healthy. Take plain yogurt or kefir

- **Eat dinner early.**

  Cut off food intake by 7 PM or 8 PM

- **Two or three times a week**

  stop taking breakfast, and break your fast with protein or do intermittent fasting

- **Take dandelion tea,**

  good for liver and other health benefits. Make dandelion salad

- **Pineapple and Papayas:** pineapples and papayas contain enzymes that aid digestion and break down proteins that usually cause bloat.

References

1. McCay CM, Crowell MF, Maynard LA. The effect of retarded growth upon the length of life span and upon the ultimate body size. Nutrition. 1935;5:155-71
2. Cheng CW, Villani V, et al. "Fasting-Mimicking Diet Promotes Ngn3-Driven β-Cell Regeneration to Reverse Diabetes." Cell. Volume 168, Issue 5, p775–788.e12, 23 February 2017
3. Cheng CW, Adams GB, et al. "Prolonged Fasting Reduces IGF-1/PKA to Promote Hematopoietic-Stem-Cell-Based Regeneration and Reverse Immunosuppression." Cell Stem Cell , Vol 14 , Issue 6 , 810 – 823
4. Ibid.
5. Emails from Dr. Sears, MD

If ypo are interested just weight loss, then try the following proven procedure:

In warm water add a couple of table spoons of apple cider vinegar (you may add raw honey according to your test) drink with **Thin Secrete Pure Garcinia Cambogia** in the morning. If you can handle vinegar without honey the better.